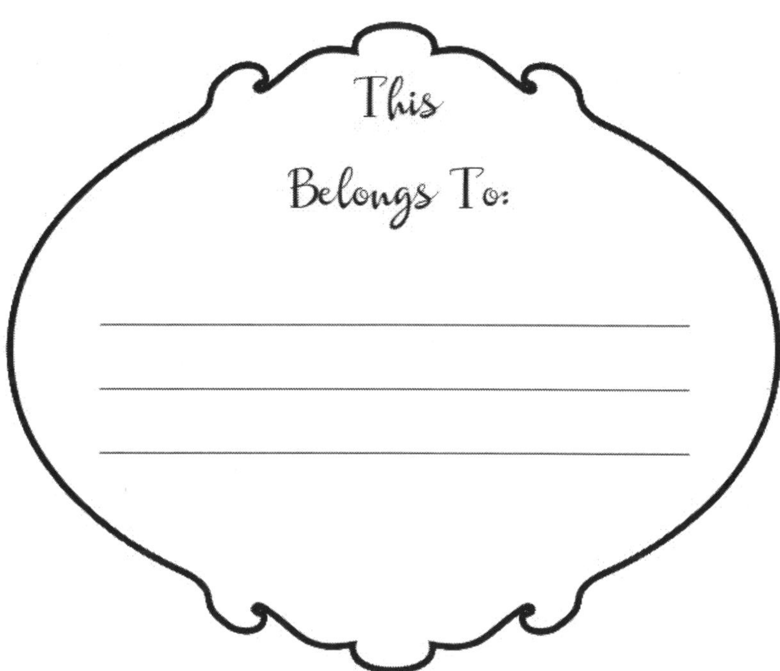
This
Belongs To:

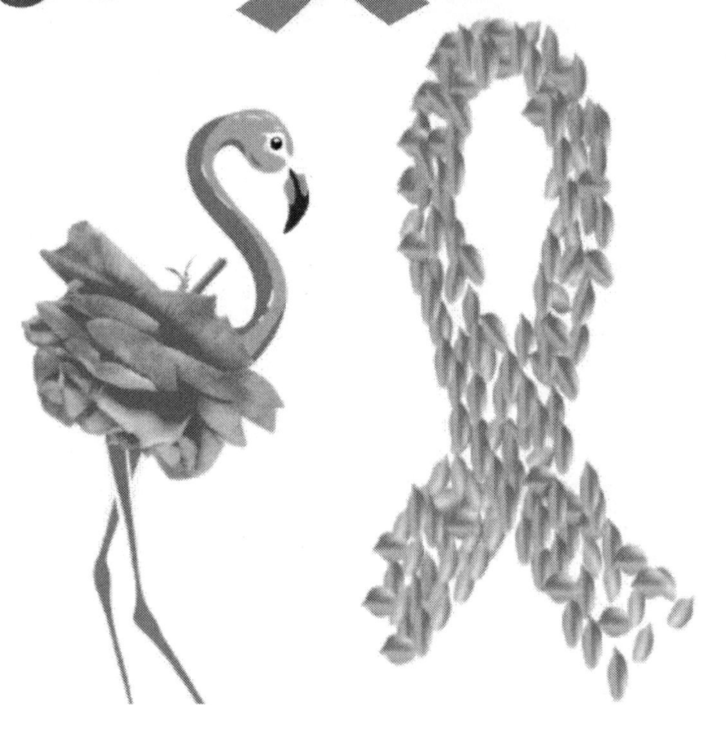
Believe

Made in the USA
Monee, IL
07 July 2026

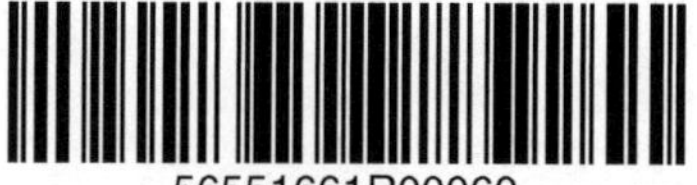